Principles of Healthcare Reimbursement

Student Workbook

SECOND EDITION

Anne B. Casto, RHIA, CCS
Elizabeth Layman, PhD, RHIA, CCS, FAHIMA

AHIMA
American Health Information Management Association®

ISBN 1-58426-207-9 or 978-1-58426-207-7
AHIMA Product No. AB332008

Ken Zielske, Director of Publications
Katie Greenock, Assistant Editor
Melissa Ulbricht, Editorial/Production Coordinator

All information contained within this book, including Web sites and regulatory information, was current and valid as of the date of publication. However, Web page addresses and the information on them may change or disappear at any time and for any number of reasons. The user is encouraged to perform his or her own general Web searches to locate any site addresses listed here that are no longer valid.

AHIMA strives to recognize the value of people from every racial and ethnic background as well as all genders, age groups, and sexual orientations by building its membership and leadership resources to reflect the rich diversity of the American population. AHIMA encourages the celebration and promotion of human diversity through education, mentoring, recognition, leadership, and other programs.

American Health Information Management Association
233 North Michigan Avenue, 21st Floor
Chicago, Illinois 60601

www.ahima.org

How To Use This Book

This workbook is intended to give students additional resources for self-study and to give professors additional resources for in-class and on-line exercises, take-home assignments, and grading opportunities.

Please do not try to use this book as a standalone text. It is written to be a companion to *Principles of Healthcare Reimbursement,* Second Edition, published by AHIMA.

Each workbook unit contains the following elements:

- Real-World Case
- Application Exercises
- Review Quiz

All pages are perforated for ease of use. Instructors are encouraged to assign students the exercises in this workbook as homework to be handed in and graded throughout the course. Answer space exists following each open-ended exercise, and an answer sheet follows each chapter's review quiz. The instructor guide contains a separate test bank with additional questions and answers for use at the instructor's discretion.

The key to all exercises is published in the instructor guide, which is available in electronic format through the Assembly on Education (AOE) Community of Practice (CoP). Instructors who are AHIMA members can sign up for this private community by clicking on the Help icon within the CoP home page and requesting additional information on becoming an AOE CoP member. An instructor who is not an AHIMA member or an AHIMA member who is not an instructor may contact the publisher at publications@ahima.org. Instructor materials also can be found on the AHIMA bookstore Web page for the textbook. The instructor materials are not available to students enrolled in college or university programs.

Chapter 1
Healthcare Reimbursement Methodologies

Elizabeth Layman, PhD, RHIA, CCS, FAHIMA

Theory into Practice

This chapter discusses concepts and definitions related to the types of healthcare reimbursement methodologies. How do actual events affect the implementation of these methodologies in U.S. society? Are healthcare reimbursement methodologies more than concepts and definitions?

Analysts studied trends in health insurance plans between the years 1993 and 2001 (Gabel, Jensen, and Hawkins 2003). These analysts found that:

- The overall percentages of workers enrolled in self-insured health plans were 55 percent in 1993, 57 percent in 1996, and 50 percent in 2001.
- The percentages of workers enrolled in various types of self-insured health plans changed over time. The percentages of workers in self-insured retrospective plans and self-insured preferred provider plans decreased between 1993 and 2001. On the other hand, the percentages of workers in self-insured health maintenance organizations increased in the time period.

Thus, between 1993 and 2001, there was an overall decrease in the percentages of workers covered by self-insured plans. The analysts attributed this decrease to the growth of managed care. Moreover, the analysts predict that, as managed care moves to less restrictive or hybrid forms, the percentages of workers in self-insured health plans will again rise.

Of particular interest is the effect of federal legislation. The Health Insurance Portability and Accountability Act (HIPAA) of 1996 prohibited the application of pre-existing condition clauses to new employees who had had health insurance prior to their employment. In effect, new employees get credit for their previous fulfillment of terms of health insurance coverage. Their credit is portable to their new employer's insurance plan. The effect of HIPAA was to greatly decrease the use of pre-existing condition clauses in health insurance policies.

Therefore, while this chapter presents information about healthcare reimbursement methodologies as concepts and definitions, these methodologies affect the decisions of human resource administrators in thousands of U.S. organizations and affect the day-to-day lives of millions of workers.

References

Gabel, Jon R., Gail A. Jensen, and Samantha Hawkins. 2003. Self-insurance in times of growing and retreating managed care. *Health Affairs* 22(2): 202–210.

Real-World Case

States have insurance commissions or state insurance departments. (See http://www.naic.org/state_web_map.htm). Generally, the missions of these commissions are to protect the public by regulating the insurance industry, by overseeing its financial transactions, and by providing assistance and information.

Many state insurance commissions provide information about Medicare's drug program. Under the Medicare Prescription Drug Improvement and Modernization Act of 2003, Medicare offered a prescription drug benefit beginning in January 1, 2006. Medicare contracted with private companies to offer Medicare-approved prescription drug cards. These private companies included pharmacies, pharmaceutical benefit management companies, fee-for-service health insurance plans, managed care plans, and preferred provider organizations. The Web sites of the state insurance departments provide links to Medicare information sheets, lists of approved companies, and tips for the selection of cards.

As other hot topics emerge, the state insurance departments respond with information and alerts. For the state health insurance departments, consumer knowledge is the best protection.

Questions

1. What is the name of your state's insurance commission?
2. What is the mission of your state's insurance commission?
3. In addition to Medicare prescription drug cards, list two consumer-related topics on the insurance commission's Web site.

Application Exercises

1. Bring a healthcare insurance card to a class session or have a healthcare insurance card at hand for an on-line discussion.
2. List all the healthcare insurance companies represented by the cards of the members of the class.
3. Is the language on the healthcare insurance cards standardized?
4. Go to the Web site of the healthcare insurance company. What are some hot topics?

Review Quiz

1. Who are the first, second, and third parties in healthcare situations?
2. Compare the UCR and CPR payment systems.
3. Describe the two purposes of managed care.
4. Why have many insurers replaced retrospective health insurance plans with group plans such as HMOs and PPOs?
5. What are advantages of capitated payments for providers and payers?
6. How do third party payers set per-diem payment rates?
7. Describe the major benefits of episode-of-care reimbursement according to its advocates and the major concerns about episode-of-care reimbursement expressed by its critics.
8. How does the payment method used by physician care groups (PCGs) account for resources used in patient care?
9. In the episode-of-care reimbursement approach, providers are reimbursed a lump sum for all provided services related to a patient's condition or disease. True or false?
10. How do clinical risk groups (CRGs) manage healthcare costs?

Chapter 2
Clinical Coding and Coding Compliance

Theory into Practice and Real World Case

The health information management team at Anywhere University Hospital (AUH) contracted with an auditing firm to perform full assessment coding review. The results from this baseline assessment are provided in four tables:

- Variation Log by Type of Error
- Variation Log by Coder
- Variation Log by MS-DRG
- MS-DRG Relationship Assessment

You are the inpatient coding manager at AUH. Your director has asked you to develop an ongoing review and monitoring schedule for the next year based on the results from the outside review.

Include internal and external reviews, coding in-services, physician workshops, and external seminars/educational sessions that will be performed and or provided for your staff. The schedule should be specific. (Include volumes and/or percentages of charts to be reviewed.) Keep in mind that on average it takes 18 minutes to review one inpatient chart. Budget provides for $15,000 for external reviews. The average cost for reviewing one inpatient record by an external review team is $45.00 (fully loaded).

In addition to preparing the schedule, outline how you will maintain coding quality statistics and report them back to the HIM Director and Compliance Committee at your facility.

How will you reward your staff members who show great improvements?

How will you reward and/or recognize that your staff has made improvements overall?

Your Coding Team consists of:
Coding Manager (you)
Data Quality Auditor (1 FTE)
8 – Inpatient Coders (8 FTE)
  2 – RHIA, CCS
  3 – CCS
  3 – RHIT

Results of the full assessment coding review for AUH
Two audits were performed:
1. Coding quality review by MS-DRG
2. MS-DRG Relationship Analysis

Variation Log by Type of Error

	% of Errors
Inaccurate sequencing or specificity principal diagnosis, affect MS-DRG	17
Inaccurate sequencing or specificity principal diagnosis, non affect MS-DRG	16
Omission CC, affect MS-DRG	33
Omission CC, non affect MS-DRG	2
Inaccurate principal procedure, affect MS-DRG	3
Omission procedure, affect MS-DRG	4
More specific coding of diagnosis or procedure, non affect MS-DRG	12
Inaccurate coding	5
Missed diagnosis or procedure code	8

Variation Log by Coder

Coder	Error Rate	Standard
Coder 1	3%	5%
Coder 2	**9%**	5%
Coder 3	**8%**	5%
Coder 4	2%	5%
Coder 5	4%	5%
Coder 6	**16%**	5%
Coder 7	**12%**	5%
Coder 8	3%	5%

Variation Log by MS-DRG*

MS-DRG	Volume	Error Rate
470	420	2%
313	233	14%
392	232	1%
291	232	17%
247	220	3%
292	216	5%
871	213	12%
641	209	0%
194	195	3%
293	193	1%
885	188	3%
312	177	0%
191	175	7%
287	173	2%
310	171	15%
689	157	11%
603	143	2%
379	137	3%
192	131	9%
683	116	11%
189	114	1%
069	110	2%
190	92	12%
193	87	10%
690	76	4%
065	76	5%
195	72	2%
066	52	2%
064	41	5%
906	35	2%

*MS-DRG descriptions provided below

Variation Log by MS-DRG* Set

MS-DRG Set	Hospital %	Nation %
064	24.3%	21.4%
065	45.0%	43.8%
066	30.8%	34.8%
190	23.1%	15.2%
191	44.0%	33.5%
192	32.9%	51.3%
193	24.6%	17.5%
194	55.1%	54.2%
195	20.3%	28.3%
291	34.6%	29.2%
292	36.7%	38.8%
293	28.8%	31.9%
689	67.4%	21.7%
690	32.6%	78.3%

*MS-DRG descriptions provided below

MS-DRG	MS-DRG Title (FY 2008)
064	Intracranial hemorrhage or cerebral infarction w MCC
065	Intracranial hemorrhage or cerebral infarction w CC
066	Intracranial hemorrhage or cerebral infarction w/o CC/MCC
069	Transient ischemia
189	Pulmonary edema & respiratory failure
190	Chronic obstructive pulmonary disease w MCC
191	Chronic obstructive pulmonary disease w CC
192	Chronic obstructive pulmonary disease w/o CC/MCC
193	Simple pneumonia & pleurisy w MCC
194	Simple pneumonia & pleurisy w CC
195	Simple pneumonia & pleurisy w/o CC/MCC
247	Perc cardiovasc proc w drug-eluting stent w/o MCC
287	Circulatory disorders except AMI, w card cath w/o MCC
291	Heart failure & shock w MCC
292	Heart failure & shock w CC
293	Heart failure & shock w/o CC/MCC
310	Cardiac arrhythmia & conduction disorders w/o CC/MCC
312	Syncope & collapse
313	Chest pain
379	G.I. hemorrhage w/o CC/MCC
392	Esophagitis, gastroent & misc digest disorders w/o MCC
470	Major joint replacement or reattachment of lower extremity w/o MCC
603	Cellulitis w/o MCC
641	Nutritional & misc metabolic disorders w/o MCC
683	Renal failure w CC
689	Kidney & urinary tract infections w/ MCC
690	Kidney & urinary tract infections w/o MCC
871	Septicemia w/o MV 96+ hours w MCC
885	Psychoses
906	Hand procedures for injuries

Application Exercises

1. Locate the current *Office of Inspector General Work Plan* on the Health and Human Services Office of Inspector General Web site. Write a memo to your Compliance Officer outlining the key areas for your inpatient facility. Identify which areas would be appropriate for the auditing schedule, which areas would be appropriate for the education schedule, and which areas would be appropriate for both schedules.

2. What is ICD-10? What is ICD-10-CM? Is this classification system important for the future of healthcare reimbursement? Why or why not?

   Begin your research with the National Center for Health Statistics Web site at: http://www.cdc.gov/nchs/.

3. Review the case mix index figures in tables 1 and 2 below. Compare the hospital figures to the state average and the peer facilities. Why are an individual hospital's figures above or below the state average? Brainstorm possible explanations for why a facility's CMI is higher or lower than the state or its peers. What MS-DRGs are included in MDC 08 that could influence changes in CMI?

Table 1—Overall CMI—Years 1–3

Facility	Year 1	Year 2	Year 3
Hospital A	1.8694	1.9017	2.1473
Hospital B	1.9662	2.0554	2.0267
Hospital C	1.6440	1.6873	1.7010
Hospital D	1.8454	1.7021	1.6250
State Average	1.4480	1.4778	1.4953

Table 2—MCD 08 CMI—Years 1–3

Facility	Year 1	Year 2	Year 3
Hospital A	1.5700	1.4941	1.3914
Hospital B	1.6917	1.8145	1.9703
Hospital C	1.7264	1.7812	1.7898
Hospital D	1.8246	1.8628	2.0187
State Average	1.5461	1.6127	1.6292

Review Quiz

Instructions: Match each coding system on the left with its description of uses on the right.

1. ICD-9-CM ___ Medical and surgical supplies
2. HCPCS Level II ___ Physician inpatient or outpatient procedures
3. CPT ___ Diagnoses and inpatient procedures

Instructions: Answer the following questions.

4. Common forms of fraud and abuse include all of the following **except:**
   a. Upcoding
   b. Unbundling
   c. Refiling claims after denials
   d. Billing for services not furnished to patients
5. Name and describe three of the seven OIG elements of an effective compliance plan.
6. Name the legislation that created Medicare Summary Notices and describe their use.
7. What is the focus of quality improvement organizations (QIOs), and how do they help to improve quality?
8. What are three target areas of the First-look Analysis Tool for Hospital Outlier Monitoring (FATHOM) software?
9. What version of the OIG Scope of Work is being used, and when will it expire?
10. What HHS tool is available for healthcare providers to use in developing coding, HIM, and corporate compliance plans?
11. For what can a manager use internal benchmarking (trending)?
12. What resource can managers use to discover current hot areas of compliance?
13. What is the primary use of a case mix index analysis?
14. How do QIOs use site-of-service reviews?
15. What payment approach has created new compliance challenges related to E/M coding of emergency department services?
16. The International Classification of Diseases (ICD) is maintained by the American Medical Association. True or false?
17. CPT Category I codes include sections for Radiology and Medicine. True or false?
18. HCPCS Level II temporary codes may be replaced with permanent codes. True or false?
19. When the 8th SOW was implemented in August 2005, the Hospital Payment Monitoring Program ended. True or false?

Chapter 3
Voluntary Healthcare Insurance Plans

Theory into Practice

Cost sharing, in the form of deductibles, copayments, coinsurance, and other out-of-pocket payments, is discussed in this chapter. But does cost sharing actually affect a healthcare consumer's bottom line, or disposable income?

In fact, over the course of a year, these outlays for healthcare can add up to a considerable sum. The Agency for Healthcare Research and Quality (AHRQ) of the U.S. Department of Health and Human Services published a research briefing enumerating these costs (Stanton 2002). Other prominent organizations, the National Coalition on Health Care, the Kaiser Family Foundation, and the Health Research and Educational Trust have, over time, compiled data and tracked trends in healthcare costs. Here are key findings from these reports:

- Average annual employer healthcare insurance premium in the private sector for single coverage was $4,479; and for family coverage,$12,106. Worker contributions were $694 and $3,281, respectively (Kaiser Family Foundation and Health Research and Educational Trust 2007, 1).
- Average annual deductibles for single coverage range from $401 to $1,729, dependent upon the type of health plan (Kaiser Family Foundation and Health Research and Educational Trust 2007, 3).
- Cost sharing, for inpatient hospital admissions, outpatient surgeries, emergency room care, physician office visits, and prescriptions, exists in addition to the annual deductibles for 95 percent of workers. For hospital inpatient admissions, this additional cost sharing is about $330 and for physician office visits about $20 (Kaiser Family Foundation and Health Research and Educational Trust 2007, 3).
- On average, per prescription copayments for brand name drugs with generic equivalents (tier 3) were $43 and for generic drugs were $11 (Kaiser Family Foundation and Health Research and Educational Trust 2007, 4).

- For people under age 65, the highest average out-of-pocket costs were for physician office visits at $104 (Stanton 2002).
- For people over the age of 65, the highest average out-of-pocket costs were for prescriptions at $397 (Stanton 2002, 7).

To help people estimate their total annual healthcare expenses, consumer services and governmental health agencies have constructed cost calculators. Subsequently, these estimates can guide consumers in their:

- Selection of healthcare plans, Medicare supplemental healthcare plans, or Medicare drug plans
- Determination of amounts of money to set aside in health savings accounts. Health savings accounts are tax-free savings accounts.

Examples of these cost calculators (estimators) are found at:

- http://www.ehealthlink.com/OregonHealthInsurance/Default.asp
- http://www.bluecrossmn.com/bc/wcs/groups/bcbsmn/@mbc_bluecrossmn/documents/public/mbc1_ps_cost_calculator.hcsp
- http://www.hsafinder.com/comparison_calculator.shtml
- http://sites.stockpoint.com/AARP/drugbenefit.asp
- The "Search Tools" page, located at http://www.medicare.gov/

As healthcare costs continue to escalate, these tools can help consumers in their daily lives.

References

Kaiser Family Foundation / Health Research and Educational Trust. 2007. Available online from http://www.kff.org/insurance/7672/index.cfm.

National Coalition on Health Care 2007 Available online from http://www.nchc.org/facts/2007%20updates/cost.pdf.

Stanton, Mark W. 2002. Reducing costs in the health care system: Learning from what has been done. *Research in Action* 9(September). Rockville, MD: Agency for Healthcare Research and Quality, Publication Number 02-0046. Available online from http://www.ahrq.gov/research/costsria/.

Real-World Case

In many states, healthcare insurance companies can refuse to cover people because of an existing or previous illness, a pre-existing condition. These people are denied healthcare insurance coverage. What happens to them?

Thirty states operate high-risk pools in order to offer healthcare insurance to people who have been denied healthcare insurance. People who are medically uninsurable often have chronic or catastrophic diseases, such as chronic kidney failure, genetic diseases, neurologic disorders, spina bifida, systemic lupus erythematosus, or transplanted organs.

State health plans are often the healthcare insurance of last resort. Many states form nonprofit associations that fund through the healthcare plan through premiums rather than tax dollars.

Analysts have studied the healthcare insurance coverage that thirty U.S. states have offered to their citizens denied healthcare insurance (Achman and Chollet 2005, Chollet 2002). These analysts found that the coverage is limited, oftentimes in ways very similar to the healthcare insurance market:

- Waiting periods for pre-existing conditions are, on average, six months.
- Annual premiums range between $1,832 and $4,920, averaging $3,083 (125 to 200 percent of state's standard rate for comparable coverage).
- Deductibles are usually $500 to $1,000, but can be as high as $10,000.
- Cost-sharing ranges between 20 and 50 percent of approved charges.
- These analysts conclude that great variation exists between the states' health plans. However, in instances where states have allocated insufficient funding or have established inadequate financing mechanisms, access to pools is curtailed because of excessively high out-of-pocket costs.

References

Achman, Lori, and Deborah Chollet. 2001. Insuring the uninsurable: An overview of state high-risk pools. Commonwealth Fund. Available online from http://www.cmwf.org/publications/publications_show.htm?doc_id=221291.

Chollet, Deborah. 2002. Expanding individual health insurance coverage: Are high-risk pools the answer? *Health Affairs—Web Exclusive* July–December: W349–W352.

Questions

1. Does your state offer healthcare insurance for high-risk patients?
2. What is the name of your state's healthcare insurance for high-risk patients?
3. What are the eligibility requirements?
4. How much are premiums, deductibles, coinsurance, and copayments?
5. What other information does the state's plan offer the state's citizens?
6. Would you be able to afford your state's healthcare insurance plan for high-risk patients?

Application Exercises

1. Bring in a healthcare insurance policy to a class session or have a healthcare insurance policy at hand for an online discussion.
2. Obtain real health bills from family members or friends. Calculate out-of-pocket costs based on the policy and the real bills.
3. Complete the table to compare and contrast the out-of-pocket costs for the policies from the healthcare insurance companies represented by class members. Add columns to the table as necessary.

Comparison: Out-of-Pocket Costs by Healthcare Insurance Company

Type of Cost	Example	Healthcare Co. A	Healthcare Co. B	Healthcare Co. C	Healthcare Co. D
Annual Premium (Monthly × 12)	\$56 × 12 = \$672 (Individual)				
Annual Deductibles	\$350 per Covered Individual				
Drugs	\$0				
Physician Office Visits	Inc. in \$350				
Inpatient	Inc. in \$350				
Outpatient	Inc. in \$350				
Mental Health	Inc. in \$350				
Outpatient Therapy (PT, OT, Speech)	Inc. in \$350				
Chiropractic	Inc. in \$350				
Other					
Copayments					
Dental	\$15 per Visit for Accident, Routine Not Covered				
Drugs	Each 34-Day Supply: \$10 Generic, \$25 Preferred Brand without Generic, \$40 Preferred Brand with Generic, \$50 Non-Preferred Brand (\$10 Generic × 12 mos. = \$120)				
Physician Office Visits	\$15 per Visit (\$15 × 4 Visits per Year = \$60)				
Inpatient	\$150 per Admission				

(Continued on next page)

Type of Cost	Example	Healthcare Co. A	Healthcare Co. B	Healthcare Co. C	Healthcare Co. D
Mental Health	$150 Inpatient Care, $15 per Visit, $100 Treatment Admission				
Outpatient Therapy (PT, OT, Speech)	$15 per Visit				
Chiropractic	$15 per Visit				
Outpatient Hospital or Amb. Surg.	$75 per Episode				
Emergency Room	$200 per Visit (Unless Admitted)				
Vision	$15 per Medical Eye Exam, Glasses etc. Not Covered				
Other					
Coinsurance	20% up to $2,000 per Member				
Inpatient	See 20% above				
Outpatient	See 20% above				
Other					
Ambulance	Prior Approval				
Home Care	Prior Approval				
Private Duty Nurse	Prior Approval				
SNF	Prior Approval				
Other Out-of-Pocket					
TOTAL	**$1,202 before Lab Work or X-rays (4 clinic visits and generic meds)**				

Review Quiz

1. What is the relation between covered conditions and covered services in private or commercial insurance plans?
2. Name at least two of the three benefit terms that mean the amount during a time-frame beyond which all covered healthcare services for an insured or dependent are paid 100 percent by the insurance plan.
3. What type of insurance policy provides benefits to: (a) a resident requiring nursing home care and services, (b) an insured who becomes blind, and (c) a homeowner who requires an eight-month recuperation after a fall down her basement stairs?
4. Why can use of a formulary be considered a policy limitation?
5. List at least three typical exclusions found in insurance plan riders.
6. Describe the health insurance plan that covers federal government employees.
7. How does Blue Cross and Blue Shield notify insureds about the extent of payments made on a claim? What data elements does that notification include?
8. Voluntary health insurance plan payments account for about one-fourth of U.S. healthcare expenditures. True or false?
9. Copayments are cost-sharing provisions of policies that require insureds to pay a flat fee to healthcare service providers and suppliers. True or false?
10. Individuals having preexisting conditions are financially better off using private healthcare plans than either employer group plans or managed care alternatives. True or false?

Chapter 4
Government-Sponsored Healthcare Programs

Theory into Practice and Real World Case

Your uncle, John Smith, is going to turn 65 in three months. He is self-employed and has owned his own homebuilding business for the past 40 years. He has purchased his own health insurance plan through an independent agent for over 20 years. Now that he will be eligible for Medicare, he wanted to know more about the program. He saw a commercial about Medicare on TV and it suggested to the viewers that they visit www.medicare.gov.

John went to the Medicare Web site, but there was so much information and unfamiliar terminology that he became frustrated and quit. He asked a few of his friends that were on Medicare how they chose their plans and they said they just signed up for the "simple plan" rather than choosing something else that "might not be quite right."

Your mother told your Uncle John that you were in a health-related major at the university, so he called you up for some advice.

Prepare a "Medicare Choices for Uncle John" grid. Your grid should be detailed and include the following: cost, deductible(s), co-payment(s), examples of covered services, and any other details you think are important. But make sure the grid is easy for Uncle John to understand. Also provide your uncle with a list of Web sites or other services that he may want to use to help him make his decision.

Application Exercises

Instructions: Complete the following assignments.

1. Medicare Part D was created by the Medicare Modernization Act of 2003. On January 1, 2006 the plan became effective. Prepare an educational session using Microsoft PowerPoint for the seniors at a nearby assisted living complex. Visit the Medicare Web site at www.medicare.gov for assistance in developing your session.

2. Compare and contrast two Medicaid plans from different states. Discuss your opinions regarding each state being able to choose how they administer the Medicaid program for their state. Does this leave some Americans at a disadvantage?

Review Quiz

1. Which program replaced the Aid to Families with Dependent Children (AFDC)?
2. What recent legislation made a substantive change to Medicare benefits, and how did they change?
3. List at least three types of Medicaid recipients required for states to qualify for federal matching funds.
4. How was the PACE venture designed to enhance the quality of life for the frail elderly population?
5. What is the target population of the State Children's Health Insurance Program (SCHIP) (Title XXI)?
6. Which TRICARE program is the most economical program for military families, and why is it less expensive than the other options?
7. What program covers healthcare costs and lost income from work-related injuries or illness of federal government employees?
8. Individuals eligible for Railroad Retirement disability or retirement benefits are ineligible for Medicare. True or false?
9. Individuals who are eligible may choose between TRICARE benefits and CHAMPVA. True or false?
10. In states having no mandated workers' compensation fund, employers must purchase insurance from private carriers or provide self-insurance coverage. True or false?

Chapter 5
Managed Care Plans

Theory into Practice

What is your recourse if your health care is denied? Consider appealing the decision.

Researchers studied the outcomes of appeals from 1998 through 2000 (Studdert and Gresenz 2003; Gresenz and Studdert 2004). The researchers abstracted information from 3,519 appeals lodged against two of the largest health maintenance organizations (HMOs) in the country. The enrollees were disputing the plans' decisions.

Of the appeals, 1,774 appeals were preservice appeals (Studdert and Gresenz 2003). Preservice denials occur before the services enrollees are seeking have been provided. The researchers classified the preservice appeals into five types: out-of-network, contractual coverage, medical necessity, administrative issue, and not evident reason. Enrollees were most likely to win appeals in cases in which the reason for the denial was not evident (52.7 percent) or which involved medical necessity (52.2 percent). Enrollees were least likely to win cases involving contractual coverage (33.2 percent). Overall, enrollees won appeals in 41.9 percent of the cases.

The researchers suggested several potential reasons for these disputes. Two striking possibilities were: (1) enrollees' beliefs that care outside the network was superior; and (2) differing interpretations of medical necessity between patients and healthcare plans.

Postservice appeals involve disputes over financial responsibility for services already obtained. Postservice appeals concerning emergency room services were the most common at these two large HMOs (Gresenz and Studdert 2004). The researchers studied 405 postservice appeals for emergency room services. The average cost of these services was $1,107. In over 90 percent of cases, enrollees won the appeal and overturned the denial. According to the plans' records, 59.8 percent of the cases were overturned based on merit, and 40.2 percent were overturned to maintain good will.

In the disputes regarding emergency services, the researchers posited that patients and healthcare plans differed in their understanding of the *prudent layperson standard.* In the prudent layperson standard, federal and state policymakers base the definition of *emergency* on a reasonable layperson's interpretation of the symptoms.

On a limited basis, denials of hospital and physician services have been studied (Greenberg et al. 2004; Isenberg 2004). On appeal, 28.9 percent of denied hospital days were overturned. Physicians who appealed $2,036.00 in denied charges were able to collect $792.47 of them upon appeal (38.9 percent).

To conclude, when denied, it is worthwhile to appeal.

References

Greenberg, Jeffrey D., Donald R. Hoover, Ranita Sharma, Helaine Noveck, Maureen Bueno, and Jeffrey L. Carson. 2004. Reimbursement denial and reversal by health plans at a university hospital. *American Journal of Medicine* 117(9):629–635.

Gresenz, Carole R., and David M. Studdert. 2004. Disputes over coverage of emergency department services: A study of two health maintenance organizations. *Annals of Emergency Medicine* 43(2):155–162.

Isenberg, Steven F. 2004. Monitoring appeal success. *Ear, Nose, and Throat Journal* 83(8):524.

Studdert, David M., and Carole R. Gresenz. 2003. Enrollee appeals of preservice coverage denials at 2 health maintenance organizations. *Journal of the American Medical Association* 289(7):864–870.

Real-World Case

Researchers studied reports of care being denied to children (Valet et al. 2004). In Tennessee, TennCare is the managed healthcare program for Medicaid recipients and uninsured individuals. Throughout Tennessee in 2002, the researchers conducted face-to-face interviews with primary caregivers of 399 children. The caregivers were asked to describe experiences with denial of care. Regarding the 399 children, 146 (36.6 percent) caregivers reported experiencing one or more denials for care in the past twelve months. Most of the children were ages one through five. Children with chronic conditions experienced a higher rate of denial than children with acute conditions.

Denials of Care by Provider

Type of Provider	Number Reporting Denials
Physician Office	50 (12.5 percent)
Dentist Office	55 (13.8 percent)
Emergency Department	8 (2.0 percent)
Pharmacy	80 (20.0 percent)
Multiple Provider Sites	45 (11.3 percent)

Many respondents perceived that they were denied care because of administrative reasons, such as the provider did not accept TennCare. However, several respondents perceived the reason to be based on reimbursement. The respondents reported being told that they would need to pay for their children's care themselves because of low reimbursement by the health plan. The researchers quoted one respondent, "The receptionist told us we had to pay. She said the office took TennCare but she wanted me to pay because TennCare is not reimbursing the dentist" (Valet et al. 2004, e38).

As a result of these denials, the respondents reported that they changed their children's physicians (51 percent) or dentists (26 percent). However, many paid for dental care out of their own pockets (17 percent). When prescriptions were denied, 26 percent appealed the denial, and 49 percent paid for the prescription. The average cost of these prescriptions was $43.71.

The respondents reported that these denials worsened their children's conditions (12 percent) or resulted in emergency room visits (16 percent). Other negative results include the children being unable to attend school (20 percent) and the caregiver needing to stay home from work with the children (14 percent).

The researchers concluded that denial of care to children is relatively common in TennCare. These denials affect children's daily lives, such as their ability to attend school, and affect other types of services, such as emergency services.

Reference

Valet, Robert S., Diane F. Kutny, Gerald B. Hickson, and William O. Cooper. 2004. Family reports of care denials for children enrolled in TennCare. *Pediatrics* 114(1):e37–e42.

Questions

1. Does your state enroll Medicaid recipients in a managed healthcare plan?
2. Have you ever been denied care?
3. TennCare provides a means to appeal a denial: http://www.tennessee.gov/tenncare/mem-appeal.html. Does your state provide a similar means?
4. TennCare provides a mechanism for enrollees to report fraud, including HMO screening: http://www.tncarefraud.tennessee.gov/. Does your state have a similar mechanism?

Application Exercises

1. Share a news story about managed care in your state or in the nation. Categorize the story as a positive, a negative, or a neutral portrayal of managed care. In class or during an online discussion, tally the numbers of positive, negative, and neutral portrayals.
2. If the previous exercise did not result in many positive news stories about MCOs, expand the search.

3. Consider tendencies of news media. Do positive stories get as much coverage? To gain the perspective of the news media, read the following article: Sherman, William. 1997. A news reporter explains his "HMO horror stories." *Managed Care* 6(9):61–64.

4. Review the appeal clauses in the policies of managed care plans. Are there common characteristics?

Review Quiz

1. Describe at least three ways in which MCOs work toward their goal of quality patient care.
2. From where do evidence-based clinical guidelines originate?
3. List at least two reasons that MCOs survey their members for feedback.
4. Name the three steps in medical necessity and utilization review.
5. Describe three types of cost controls used by MCOs.
6. Which type of HMO offers patients the least selection in referrals to specialists?
7. List at least five types of services or populations that are common examples of carve outs.
8. Disease management is closely associated with coordination of care tools of MCOs because efforts of multiple providers must be synchronized in disease management. True or false?
9. Integrated delivery systems typically have horizontal rather than vertical integration of services. True or false?
10. The least binding degree of healthcare service integration is affiliation, and the highest degree of integration is the merger. True or false?

Chapter 6
Medicare-Medicaid Prospective Payment Systems for Inpatients

Theory into Practice and Real World Case

The Medicare Provider Analysis and Review (MedPAR) file is a database that the Centers for Medicare and Medicaid Services maintains. For each year, it includes the records from all the claims for hospital discharges of Medicare beneficiaries. The MedPAR file contains several gigabytes of data per year. Rather than being an inert archive, these data can be used to improve the quality of care for Medicare beneficiaries (Ash et al. 2003; Stringham and Young 2005).

The MedPAR file is an administrative database. The data include many administrative fields, such as diagnosis and procedure codes, claim costs and charges, the diagnosis related group (DRG) and as of FY08, MS-DRGs, and the length of stay. However, as an administrative database, it has limitations as a means of assessing the quality of patient care. The database does not include some clinical risk factors, such as the results of diagnostic tests. The number of other diagnoses used to record complications and comorbidities is restricted to eight. The benefits of using the database, though, far outweigh the limitations. Cost is minimal. The database already exists. No forms or procedures need to be created. No data collectors need to be hired nor trained. Data collection occurs in the usual course of business. Finally, though, research has found that the MedPAR file can be used to assess the quality of patient care for both Medicare patients and other-payer patients (Needleman et al. 2003).

Arlene Ash and colleagues used MedPAR claims data to predict mortality in patients who had suffered acute myocardial infarction (AMI). They studied the years 1995 through 1999 with more than 300,000 cases per year (305,468; 308,997; 306,224; 304,882; 306,175; totaling 1,531,7460). The validation data showed up to 80 percent mortality one year post-AMI for cases in the highest risk group. Moreover, the authors found that, prior to the AMI in the study, the patients had had a previous AMI, diabetes, or congestive heart failure. This information about health status at admission is important for the care of patients and for the improvement of care outcomes.

Stringham and Young used the MedPAR file to examine rates of urinary tract infections (UTI) at acute inpatient hospitals (2005). The authors noted that Medicare makes additional payments for complications, even complications that are possibly preventable. The relative weights of the DRGs with the complication comorbidity (CC) or major complication comorbidity (MCC) are higher than the relative weight for the DRG without the CC or MCC.

Nosocomial UTIs are an example of a potentially preventable complication. The authors explained that more expensive anti-infective catheters and staff training can reduce the rate of nosocomial UTIs.

The authors' study was designed as follows:

- All patients discharged during October 1, 2001 through September 30, 2002 as reported in the MedPAR file
- Identification of all cases with ICD-9-CM codes of 599.0 (urinary tract infection) or 996.64 (infection and inflammatory reaction due to indwelling urinary catheter)
- Elimination of cases in which urinary tract infection was the principal diagnosis or in which the Major Diagnostic Category was 18 (Infectious and Parasitic Diseases).

The total cases that resulted with qualifying UTIs were 1,012,041 of the 12,502,700 discharges. For the 1,000 hospitals with the most discharges in the MedPAR data set, the rate of secondary UTI ranged from 3.10 percent to 15.49 percent.

The authors examined the cases of one New York hospital in detail. They found that the hospital received approximately $675,000 more in Medicare payments because of the nosocomial UTIs. The more expensive, anti-infective catheters would have cost approximately $50,000. The authors hypothesized that payment policies of the Centers for Medicare and Medicaid Services (CMS) discouraged the implementation of initiatives to reduce nosocomial complications. Finally, the authors concluded that patients would benefit from improved quality of healthcare if the CMS ceased paying extra for nosocomial infections.

The MedPAR file is a valuable tool to study the quality of patient care. Therefore, besides being an abstract payment system for some people, Medicare's prospective payment system affects the health of all of us.

References

Ash, Arlene S., Michael A. Posner, Jeanne Speckman, Shakira Franco, Andrew C. Yacht, and Lindsey Bramwell. 2003. Using claims data to examine mortality trends following hospitalization for heart attack in Medicare. *Health Services Research* 38(5):1253–1262.

Needleman, Jack, Peter I. Buerhaus, Soeren Mattke, Maureen Stewart, and Katya Zelevinsky. 2003. Measuring hospital quality: Can Medicare data substitute for all-payer data? *Health Services Research* 38 (6 Part 1):1487–1508.

Stringham, Jerry, and Nancy Young. 2005. Using MedPAR data as a measure of urinary tract infection rates: Implications for the Medicare inpatient DRG payment system. *Perspectives in Health Information Management* 2(12):1–14.

Application Exercises

1. SNF: What rates and indexes must be obtained from the *Federal Register* to calculate a federal wage-adjusted SNF payment? What is the date of the most recent *Federal Register* that provides these data? After January 1, 2008, what are the SNF PPS payments for 135 days of care:
   a. At refined RUG III category RUB?
   b. At refined RUG III category IB2?
2. LTCH: To calculate unadjusted LTCH-PPS payments, what data must be obtained from the most current *Federal Register*? What is the date of the most recent *Federal Register* that provides these data? Calculate the unadjusted payments for the following cases:
   a. MS-LTC DRG = 207, Respiratory system diagnosis with ventilator support 96+ hours
   b. The patient suffered a right-sided middle cerebral artery (MCA) thrombotic occlusion with impairment (ICD-9-CM 434.01). The patient was admitted to the acute care hospital with left severe hemiplegia, left hemianesthesia, homonymous hemianopia, and aphasia. The patient's hemianopia resolved late in the admission.

      The patient was discharged from the acute care hospital and then admitted to a long-term care facility for further treatment of left-sided hemiplegia (ICD-9-CM 438.20, Late effects of cerebrovascular disease, hemiplegia affecting unspecified side), hemianesthesia (ICD-9-CM 438.6, Late effects of cerebrovascular disease, alterations of sensations; ICD-9-CM 782.0, Disturbance of skin sensation), and aphasia (ICD-9-CM 438.11, Late effects of cerebrovascular disease, aphasia). The principal diagnosis for the LTCH was the hemiplegia resulting in the MS-LTC-DRG of 056, Degenerative nervous system disorders with MCC.

3. IRF: Review the *Federal Register* for the past three years. Complete the table below.

	2 Years Ago	1 Year Ago	Current Year
Year			
Local Wage Index			
Standard Payment Conversion Factor			
Impact of Change in Wage Index (+ or –) Per Case			
Multiplied by No. of Discharges Annually (Ex: 370)			

a. For an inpatient rehabilitation facility (IRF) with 370 discharges annually, calculate the three years' partially adjusted payment rates using both the wage indexes and the standard payment conversion factors.

b. For an inpatient rehabilitation facility IRF with 370 discharges annually, calculate the three years' partially adjusted payment rates, holding the local wage index constant (only use the local wage index from "2 years ago") and using the updated standard payment conversion factor for each year.

c. For an inpatient rehabilitation facility IRF with 370 discharges annually, calculate the three years' partially adjusted payment rates, using the updated local wage index for each year and holding the standard payment conversion factor constant (only use the standard payment conversion factor from "2 years ago").

d. What are the impacts of changes in the local wage index of the student's geographic area and the standard payment conversion factor? What actions would you expect the leadership of the IRF to take?

4. IPF PPS: Use the information found in figures 1–2 (below) and tables 6.25–6.29 from the textbook to complete table 1 in order to determine the IPFPPS reimbursement for this encounter.

Figure 1: Facility Information

Bed size: 350 beds	Location: Columbus, Ohio
Classification: Rural	Wage Index: .9806
Full Service ED: Yes	Per-diem unadjusted rate: $614.99

Figure 2: Claim Information

Admit Date: January 1, 2008	Discharge Date: January 15, 2008	LOS: 14 days
Patient Age: 62		
Principal Diagnosis: 295.34	Paraphrenic schizophrenia, chronic with acute exacerbation	
Secondary Diagnosis: 301.6	Dependent personality disorder	
Secondary Diagnosis: 250.02	Uncontrolled diabetes mellitus	
MS-DRG: 885	Psychoses	
ECT treatments: 90870	3 units	$264.77 per unit

IPF PPS Payment Determination Steps

Step One:	Wage index adjust the labor portion of the per-diem rate
Step Two:	Apply COLA to the nonlabor portion of the per-diem rate if applicable
Step Three:	Add results of step one and step two to determine the wage adjusted per-diem rate
Step Four:	Apply the patient-level and facility-level adjustments
Step Five:	Multiply the PPS adjustment factor by the wage adjusted per-diem rate to calculate the adjusted per-diem rate
Step Six:	Identify whether the facility has a qualifying ED.
Step Seven:	Multiply the adjusted per-diem rate by the LOS adjustment factor for each day of the stay to calculate the per-diem payment amount
Step Eight:	Sum the per-diem payment amounts calculated for each day of stay
Step Nine:	Calculate the adjusted ECT amount if applicable
Step Ten:	Sum payments to calculate IPFPPS reimbursement

Table 1

Step	Methodology	Total
One	(per-diem rate × .75788 × WI)	
Two	If COLA then (per-diem rate ×.24212 × COLA) If non-COLA then (per-diem rate × .24212)	
Three	Sum results of step 1 and step 2	
Four	Use mini-worksheet A (see below)	
Five	Multiply result of step 3 times result of step 4	
Six	If full service ED then choose higher Day 1 adjustment in step 7 If not full service ED then choose lower Day 1 adjustment in step 7	
Seven	Use mini-worksheet B (see below)	
Eight	Sum of day rates calculated in step 7	
Nine	If COLA then ((ECT pymt rate × .75788 × WI)+(ECT pymt rate × .24212 × COLA)) × units of service If non-COLA then ((ECT pymt rate × .75788 × WI) + (ECT pymt rate × .24212)) × units of service	
Ten	Sum results of step 8 and 9	

Mini Worksheet A			
Step Four	A. Enter adjustment factor if rural location:		Enter PPS adjustment factor in Table 1 row four.
	B. Enter adjustment factor if teaching facility:		
	C. Enter adjustment factor for DRG:		
	D. Enter adjustment factor for comorbidity:		
	E. Enter adjustment factor for age:		
	Multiply applicable adjustment factors together to determine PPS adjustment factor:		

Mini Worksheet B			
Step Seven	**Day**	**Adjustment Factor**	**Adj. Factor × adjusted per-diem rate (step 5)**
	Day one		
	Day two		
	Day three		
	Day four		
	Day five		
	Day six		
	Day seven		
	Day eight		
	Day nine		
	Day ten		
	Day eleven		
	Day twelve		
	Day thirteen		
	Day fourteen		

5. IPPS: Each year new and innovative devices are considered for the new Technology add-on payment provision under IPPS. The Safe-Cross®, radio frequency total occlusion crossing system, was considered for add-on payment for FY 2006 (*Federal Register* 70(155):47359–61). Even though Safe-Cross® was not granted new technology add-on status, it is still used for many patients.

   The Safe-Cross® guidewire is present on the following claim. Complete an outlier payment calculation to determine if this claim would qualify for a high cost outlier payment. If the claim qualifies for outlier payment, calculate the total reimbursement for this claim, including the additional amount that the facility would receive for the high cost outlier.

   The FY 2008 IPPS high-cost outlier threshold is $22,185.00; the hospital-specific CCR is .329; the hospital base rate is $5,200.00

Inpatient Claim		
Admit Date: January 1, 2008	Discharge Date: January 10, 2008	Length of Stay: 9 days
Principal Diagnosis:	410.71	Subendocardial infarction, initial episode of care
Secondary Diagnosis:	414.01	Coronary atherosclerosis of native coronary artery
Secondary Diagnosis:	427.1	Paroxysmal ventricular tachycardia
Secondary Diagnosis:	272.0	Pure hypercholesterolemia
Principal Procedure:	00.66	Percutaneous transluminal coronary angioplasty
Secondary Procedure:	36.07	Insertion of drug-eluting coronary artery stent
Secondary Procedure:	39.29	Other vascular shunt or bypass
Secondary Procedure:	37.22	Left heart cardiac catheterization
DRG: 246 RW: 2.8717	Percutaneous cardiovascular procedure with drug-eluting stent with MCC or 4+ vessels/stents	

Claim Detail		
Revenue Code	**Revenue Code Description**	**Charge**
110	Room & board—private	$4,375.00
120	Room & board—semi private	$1,700.00
200	Intensive care—general	$2,910.00
206	Intensive care—intermediate ICU	$1,780.00
250	Pharmacy—general	$1,486.66
255	Pharmacy—drugs incident to radiology	$728.13
258	Pharmacy—IV solutions	$1,583.60
259	Pharmacy—other pharmacy	$7,766.18
270	Medical/surgical supplies—general	$8,256.00
272	Medical/surgical supplies—sterile supply	$8,366.25
272	The Safe-Cross® guidewire	$12,000.00
278	Medical/surgical supplies—other implants	$28,623.00
301	Laboratory—chemistry	$2,739.00
302	Laboratory—Immunology	$648.00
305	Laboratory—Hematology	$2,335.00
323	Laboratory—Arteriography	$2,491.00
360	Operating room—general	$13,875.00
361	Operating room—minor surgery	$517.00
370	Anesthesia—general	$209.00
390	Blood and blood component admin, process, storage—gen	$668.00
410	Respiratory services—general	$21.00
420	Physical therapy—general	$314.00
430	Occupational therapy—general	$441.00
480	Cardiology—general	$5,629.00
481	Cardiology—cardiac cath lab	$6,249.00
483	Cardiology—echocardiology	$1,786.00
710	Recovery room—general	$1,648.00
730	EKG/ECG—general	$1,098.00
921	Other diagnostic services—peripheral vascular lab	$359.00
	TOTAL CHARGE:	$120,601.80

6. IPPS: The top 25 MS-DRGs for Hospital A are provided in the table below. Calculate the case mix index for this MS-DRG set.

MS-DRG	MS-DRG Title	Volume	MDC	TYPE	RW
470	Major joint replacement or reattachment of lower extremity w/o MCC	420	08	SUR	1.9871
392	Esophagitis, gastroent & misc digest disorders w/o MCC	332	06	MED	0.7120
194	Simple pneumonia & pleurisy w CC	295	04	MED	1.0234
247	Perc cardiovasc proc w drug-eluting stent w/o MCC	280	05	SUR	2.1254
293	Heart failure & shock w/o CC/MCC	246	05	MED	0.8764
313	Chest pain	233	05	MED	0.5488
292	Heart failure & shock w CC	232	05	MED	1.0133
690	Kidney & urinary tract infections w/o MCC	219	11	MED	0.8000
192	Chronic obstructive pulmonary disease w/o CC/MCC	218	04	MED	0.8144
871	Septicemia w/o MV 96+ hours w MCC	213	18	MED	1.7483
641	Nutritional & misc metabolic disorders w/o MCC	209	10	MED	0.7248
291	Heart failure & shock w MCC	193	05	MED	1.2585
885	Psychoses	188	19	MED	0.7783
312	Syncope & collapse	177	05	MED	0.7197
287	Circulatory disorders except AMI, w card cath w/o MCC	173	05	MED	1.1412
195	Simple pneumonia & pleurisy w/o CC/MCC	172	04	MED	0.8397
310	Cardiac arrhythmia & conduction disorders w/o CC/MCC	171	05	MED	0.6438
603	Cellulitis w/o MCC	143	09	MED	0.8086
379	G.I. hemorrhage w/o CC/MCC	137	06	MED	0.8475
191	Chronic obstructive pulmonary disease w CC	131	04	MED	0.9405
065	Intracranial hemorrhage or cerebral infarction w CC	128	01	MED	1.1900
683	Renal failure w CC	116	11	MED	1.1941
189	Pulmonary edema & respiratory failure	114	04	MED	1.36605
069	Transient ischemia	110	01	MED	0.7339
066	Intracranial hemorrhage or cerebral infarction w/o CC/MCC	102	01	MED	1.0302

Review Quiz

1. List at least two major reasons that Medicare administrators turned to the prospective payment concept for Medicare beneficiaries.
2. How do DRGs encourage inpatient facilities to practice cost management?
3. How are per-diem rates for SNF PPS patients determined for various cases?
4. How are MS-LTC-DRGs determined?
5. On the IRF PAI the patient's ability to perform activities of daily living, or _____ is recorded on the _____.
6. Why does the IPF PPS length-of-stay adjustment factor grow smaller during the patient encounter?
7. Describe at least two of the patient-level adjustments for IRF PPS claims and why they are used.
8. For inpatient rehabilitation facility patients, codes on the IRF PAI should follow the UHDDS and the UB-04 guidelines. True or false?
9. Facilities transmit IRF PAIs to the Centers for Medicare and Medicaid Services using CMS's free IRVEN software. True or false?

Chapter 7
Ambulatory and Other Medicare-Medicaid Reimbursement Systems

Theory into Practice and Real-World Case

Third party payers have adopted Medicare's resource-based relative value scale (RBRVS). Because of its widespread use, the RBRVS has been suggested as a means of financial analysis (Melzer et al. 2001; Melzer, Richards, and Covington 2004; Rotarius and Liberman 2001).

Melzer and colleagues used the RBRVS to analyze the viability of a pediatric hospitalist program (2001). The researchers reviewed one year of discharge and billing data from a 208-bed children's hospital. Key data in their evaluation were:

- Relative value units for the three levels of initial hospital care and subsequent hospital care
- Conversion factor
- Actual physician salaries
- Average daily census of the unit

During the period of the study (July 1997 through June 1998), the RVUs ranged from 1.04 through 4.29, the conversion factor was $24.46, and the average daily census was 7.2 patients.

The researchers examined various scenarios of salaries, average daily census, conversion factors, and operating expenses. For this specific pediatric unit, the researchers concluded that the revenue generated was inadequate to support the physicians' salaries and operating expenses for the time spent attending the patients. To cover these costs, either the average daily census needed to increase to 9 patients or the conversion factor needed to increase to $31. The researchers suggested that their process can be a model to financially evaluate other hospitalist programs.

Researchers also examined whether the RBRVS payment method sufficiently covered the expenses of a multidisciplinary team treating pediatric ambulatory diabetes patients in a pediatric endocrinology and diabetes clinic (Melzer, Richards, and Covington 2004). The researchers explained that ambulatory pediatric care for diabetes mellitus has evolved to a multidisciplinary team approach. The team comprises pediatric endocrinologists, certified diabetes mellitus nurse educators, nurse practitioners, dieticians, social workers, and psychologists. The clinic receives one payment based on the RBRVS for these complex services.

To study the adequacy of the reimbursement for multidisciplinary care, billing data and financial income and expense reports for the period July 1, 2003 through June 30, 2001 were reviewed. The researchers found that 30 percent (1420) of the patient visits were for care of diabetes mellitus. The clinic followed the recommendations of the American Diabetes Association for optimal case management. These recommendations include patient and family education; managing daily insulin injections, diet, and exercise; and long-term monitoring. The researchers noted that the telephone management of glycemic control was particularly expensive, although an important component of care.

The researchers calculated revenue using the RBRVS method. They found that revenues generated under the RBRVS method were sufficient for the physicians' expenses in the team approach. However, the researchers found that the revenues generated under the RBRVS method only covered 16 percent of the actual nonphysician practice expenses in the multidisciplinary model. Thus, the reimbursement does not adequately reimburse the clinic for the nonphysician and facility practice expenses. The researchers concluded that the multidisciplinary care model may not be financially viable.

Rotarius and Liberman concluded that analysis using the RBRVS provides valuable information. The types of information include:

- Fulfillment of contractual payment rates by healthcare insurance plans
- Profitability of specific procedures
- Optimal mix of physician specialties
- Projections for contract negotiations

Therefore, analysis using the RBRVS is a means of financial management and strategic planning.

A student in a health services management (HSM) academic program was serving as an intern in a physician practice. The student had read the previous articles about the potential for insufficient reimbursements under the RBRVS payment method. The HSM intern decided to analyze the financial viability of the practice. The intern compiled the following spreadsheet:

Any Year: Projected Revenue by CPT® Visit Code*

Item	Work RVU	Non-Fac PE RVU	MP RVU	Tot RVU (Col B + Col C + Col D)	Conversion Factor $36.177	Number Annually	Projected Revenue (Col E × Col F × Col G)
99202—Office Visit, New, Straightforward Medical Decision Making	0.88	0.79	0.05	1.72		45	$2,800.10
99203—Office Visit, New, Low Complexity Medical Decision Making	1.34	1.13	0.09	2.56		50	$4,630.66
99204—Office Visit, New, Moderate Complexity Medical Decision Making	2.00	1.50	0.12	3.62		120	$15,715.29
99205—Office Visit, New, High Complexity Medical Decision Making	2.67	1.78	0.15	4.60		360	$59,909.11
99211—Office Visit, Est., May Not Require Presence of Physician	0.17	0.39	0.01	0.57		100	$2,062.09
99212—Office Visit, Est., Straightforward Medical Decision Making	0.45	0.54	0.03	1.02		500	$18,450.27
99213—Office Visit, Est., Low Complexity Medical Decision Making	0.67	0.69	0.03	1.39		600	$30,171.62
99214—Office Visit, Est., Moderate Complexity Medical Decision Making	1.10	1.03	0.05	2.18		4600	$362,782.96
99215—Office Visit, Est., High Complexity Medical Decision Making	1.77	1.32	0.08	3.17		2000	$229,362.18
						8375	$725,884.27

*Values are representative only; readers are cautioned to check current *Federal Register* and CPT®.

References

Melzer, Sanford M., Richard A. Molteni, Edgar K. Marcuse, and Frederick P. Rivara. 2001. Characteristics and financial performance of a pediatric faculty inpatient attending service: A resource-based relative value scale analysis. *Pediatrics* 108(1):79–84.

Melzer, Sanford M., Gail E. Richards, and Maxine L. Covington. 2004. Reimbursement and costs of pediatric ambulatory diabetes care by using the resource-based relative value scale: Is multidisciplinary care financially viable? *Pediatric Diabetes* 5(3):133–142.

Rotarius, Timothy, and Aaron Liberman. 2001. An RBRVS approach to financial analysis in health care organizations. *Health Care Manager* 19(3):17–23.

Questions

1. What factors other than financial performance can leaders of healthcare organizations consider as they evaluate organizational programs?
2. What reasons could account for the gap between the reimbursement for multidisciplinary care and the expenses of delivery of multidisciplinary care?
3. In evaluating the RBRVS reimbursements for the physician practice, what other data should the intern consider? The intern notes that code 99205 has the highest RVU. Explain whether the intern should advise the practice to recruit more very sick new patients (Office visit, new patient, high complexity).

Application Exercises

1. Resource-Based Relative Value Scale (RBRVS): For the previous year and current year, obtain the necessary data from the *Federal Register* and from the Web site of the Centers for Medicare and Medicaid Services (Physician Fee Schedule Look-up, Physician Fee Schedule Search) to calculate Medicare reimbursement payments under the RBRVS method. Calculate the reimbursements under the RBRVS method for the previous year and the current year for the following CPT® codes:
   a. 31239
   b. 68720
   c. 68815

   Are there any unique data, such as the budget neutrality (BN) adjustor in 2007, that must be obtained? What factor has had the greatest impact on reimbursement for each procedure? If profit were the physician's only motive, in which site would procedure 68815 be performed? What factors other than reimbursement do physicians consider when they select the site of a procedure?
2. Ambulance Fee Schedule: In February, 2007, via CMS transmittal R1185CP, CMS introduced a revised Medical Conditions List to the Ambulance Fee Schedule. Download this transmittal from the CMS Web site and prepare an education presentation.

Include the importance of the Medical Conditions List, how the list should be used, and any precautions that ambulance suppliers should take when using this list to determine the appropriate level of service.

3. Home Health PPS: The unit of payment in the home health prospective payment system is the episode of care.
   a. How does Medicare define an episode of care for home health patients?
   b. Using the table below, calculate home health payments for a case with a weight of 1.9413 in two urban areas: Abilene, Texas, and Anchorage, Alaska.

Weight 1.9413	Nat'l 60-day episode rate (CY current) ($)	Unadjusted rate ($)	Labor-related ratio	Local wage index	Adj labor portion (unadj. rate × labor ratio × local wage index)	Non-labor related ratio	Unadjusted nonlabor portion (unadj. rate × nonlabor ratio)	Wage adj. rate (adj. labor portion + unadj. nonlabor ratio) ($)

   What are the CBSA codes for the two urban areas?

   How much difference do the varying local wage indexes make in the wage adjusted rate?

   c. As discussed in the text, Medicare adjusts the episode-of-care payment method when a home health agency provides four or fewer visits in an episode. The adjustment is called a low-utilization payment adjustment (LUPA). Under LUPA, Medicare pays the national per-visit amount by discipline. Check the most recent *Federal Register* for the current national per-visit amounts by discipline. Record your findings on the table that follows:

National Per-Visit Amounts for LUPAs by Discipline (Not Including A Beneficiary's Only Episode or the Initial Episode in a Sequence of Adjacent Episodes)*

Home Health Discipline Type	Per-Visit Payment Amount CY Current Year
Home Health Aide	
Medical Social Services	
Occupational Therapy	
Physical Therapy	
Skilled Nursing	
Speech-Language Pathology	

*Modified Source: *Federal Register* 70(216):68134.

Department of Health and Human Services. 2005 (November 9). Medicare Program; Home Health Prospective Payment System Rate Update for Calendar Year 2006; Final Rule. *Federal Register* 70(216):68132–68215.

4. HOPPS/ASC: Use the information found in figures 1–5 below to complete tables 1 and 2 and determine the HOPPS and ASC reimbursement rates for a cataract procedure. Answer the short discussion question.

Figure 1: Hospital Information

Bed size: 300 beds	**Teaching status:** Nonteaching	**Wage index: .9971**
Cost to Charge Ratios (CCRs)		
RC 250	Pharmacy, general	0.408344
RC 270	Supplies, general	0.796788
RC 271	Nonsterile supply	0.796788
RC 272	Sterile supply	0.796788
RC 276	Intraocular lens	0.796788
RC 301	Chemistry	0.291546
RC 312	Pathology, surgical	0.291546
RC 360	Operating room	0.404314
RC 370	Anesthesia	0.321246
RC 710	Recovery room	0.404314
RC 730	EKG	0.38251
RC 920	Diagnostic services	0.88447

Figure 2: Claim Information Hospital Outpatient Department

Admit date 2/20/2008	Discharge date 2/20/2008		
Sex: F Age: 70 LOS: 1 day			
Admit diagnosis	366.9	Cataract, unspecified	
Principal diagnosis:	366.10	Senile cataract, unspecified	
Principal procedure:	66984	Cataract extraction with IOL insertion	
Charge Detail			
Revenue Code	**CPT/HCPCS Code**	**Code Description**	**Charge**
250			$475.25
270			$280.25
271			$1178.18
272			$1297.07
276			$351.00
301	36415	Routine venipuncture	$10.00
301	82565	Assay of creatinine	$33.75
301	84132	Assay of serum potassium	$33.75
301	85014	Hematocrit	$34.75
312	88304	Tissue exam by pathologist	$83.50
360	66984	Cataract extraction w/IOL	$801.33
370			$574.00
710			$341.00
730	93005	Electrocardiogram, tracing	$124.50
920	90772	Ther/proph/diag inj, sc/im	$75.50
		TOTAL Charges	$5,693.83
		Medicare beneficiary copayment amount:	$516.79

Figure 3: Claim Information Ambulatory Surgery Center

CPT Code: 66984	**Cataract extraction with IOL**	**Charges: $2,500.00**
	Medicare beneficiary copayment amount:	$197.61

Figure 4: Fee Schedule Information

Revenue Code	CPT/HCPCS	Fee Schedule Amt	Status Indicator
301	36415	$3.00	A
301	82565	$7.07	A
301	84132	$6.35	A
301	85014	$3.27	A

Figure 5: APC Information

Revenue Code	CPT Code	APC	Relative Weight	Status Indicator
312	88304	0343	.5142	X
360	66984	0246	23.8649	T
730	93005	0099	.3892	S
920	90772	0437	.3945	S

HOPPS Payment Determination Steps

Step One: Calculate APC payment rate(s)
Step Two: Wage index adjust APCs
Step Three: Sum of fees for status indicator A procedures
Step Four: Sum of reasonable cost amount(s) (status indicators L and H)
Step Five: Sum Medicare payments

Table 1

Step	Methodology	Total
One	APC relative weight × conversion factor ($63.694)	
Two	(APC pymt rate × .60×WI) + (APC pymt rate × .40)	
Three	Fee schedule amount A + fee schedule amount B, etc.	
Four	(Charge × CCR)	
Five	Total Reimbursement – Sum of steps 2–4	

ASC Payment Determination Steps

Step One: Calculate APC payment rate(s)
Step Two: Wage index adjust APCs
Step Three: Calculate the APC payment rate for any allowed secondary procedures
Step Four: Wage index adjust allowed secondary procedure APCs
Step Five: Sum Medicare payments

Table 2

Step	Methodology	Total
One	APC relative weight × conversion factor ($41.401)	
Two	(APC pymt rate × .50*WI) + (APC pymt rate × .50)	
Three	APC relative weight × conversion factor ($41.401)	
Four	(APC pymt rate × .50*WI) + (APC pymt rate × .50)	
Five	TOTAL Reimbursement – Sum of steps 2–4	

Short Discussion Question

Discuss the parity/disparity between the payment levels at the ASC and Hospital-based surgery center. Why is parity/disparity an important topic to discuss? How does it affect the average Medicare beneficiary?

Review Quiz

1. How can physician payments be adjusted for the price differences among various parts of the country?
2. What is the control mechanism the government uses on Medicare payments to physicians and how is it applied?
3. Describe at least two issues that delayed implementation of the APC system for ambulatory surgical centers.
4. What is the current status of the ASC PPS?
5. How is the two-times rule applied to APC groups?
6. In the HHPPS, the _____ software is used to collect and submit OASIS data.
7. How is durable medical equipment (DME) reimbursed in the HHPPS?
8. When a patient is pronounced dead during ambulance transport, Medicare payment rules are followed as if the patient were alive. True or false?
9. CMS, not the APC Advisory Panel or MedPAC, makes the final ruling for updates and changes to HOPPS. True or false?
10. The number of APCs per encounter for a single patient is limited to ten. True or false?

Chapter 8
Revenue Cycle Management

Theory into Practice and Real-World Case

Anywhere Hospital's CFO for the past 20 years, Jim Smith, just retired. He worked for the hospital for 40 years and was greatly respected by his staff. The hospital governing board has hired a new CFO, Todd White.

Jim Smith utilized the silo approach to revenue cycle management during his tenure. He relied on his key management personnel to contact upper management of other departments in the hospital to discuss issues and to resolve problems and vice versa.

Todd White, however, had implemented an integrated revenue cycle team at his former hospital three years ago and strongly believed in the power of teamwork. His previous team had gained numerous efficiencies and improved accounts receivable by millions. So when Todd started at Anywhere Hospital he planned on implementing a similar revenue cycle team.

As with any change, Todd was met with much resistance. But after speaking with many of his managers in patient accounts and finance, he realized that the employees did not know how to effectively work in teams because the previous CFO had not asked them to do so in several years.

Questions

1. What are some creative ways that Todd can help Anywhere Hospital understand the importance of an integrated revenue cycle team?
2. How can a manager improve teamwork amongst his/her employees?
3. Does Todd need assistance from a change management leader? Explain your answer.

Application Exercise

1. Each year CMS publishes a listing of all new technologies eligible for the new technology add-on payment provision in the *Federal Register*. Below is a listing of the devices eligible for the new technology add-on payment for FY 2006.

   Kinetra Implantable Neurostimulator for Deep Brain Stimulation
   Used for: Parkinson's disease & essential tremor
   Cost = \$16,570
   Payment up to \$8,285

   Endovascular Graft Repair of Thoracic Aorta (GORE TAG)
   Used for: management of descending thoracic aortic aneurysms
   Cost = \$21,198
   Payment up to \$10,599

   Restore Rechargeable Implantable Neurostimulator
   Used for: chronic intractable pain (blocks pain)
   Cost = \$18,640
   Payment up to \$9,320

   You are the CDM Coordinator at Anywhere Hospital. Answer the following questions about the new technology add-on payment items/devices for FY 2006.

   a. When would these items/devices be incorporated into the CDM?

   b. How would these items/devices be incorporated into the CDM?

   c. Which departments/units within Anywhere Hospital would you provide educational sessions?

   d. How would you explain the importance of the new technology add-on payment to various department/unit managers?

   Note: For CY 2008 there are no add-on new technologies. However, it is important that students understand this provision of IPPS. Therefore this application exercise is included in the workbook even though it is for CY 2006 items.

2. Read the article *Diagnosis Coding and Medical Necessity: Rules and Reimbursement* by Janis Cogley located in Appendix B of the textbook.

   This article discusses how Medicare Carriers and Fiscal Intermediaries use coverage determinations to establish medical necessity. When the condition(s) of a patient are expected to not meet medical necessity requirements for a test, procedure, or service, the provider has the obligation under the Beneficiary Notices Initiative to alert the Medicare beneficiary prior to rendering the service. The Medicare beneficiary is notified via the Advance Beneficiary Notice (ABN) (see page 235 in Appendix B).

   The Medicare beneficiary may choose to complete the ABN and provide out-of-pocket reimbursement for the service, or may elect to not have the service performed.

If the provider fails to alert the Medicare beneficiary with an ABN, then the facility may not balance bill the patient for the noncovered charges denied by the Medicare Carrier or FI.

Scenario:

You are the Revenue Cycle Coordinator for Anywhere Hospital. The Decision Support department at Anywhere Hospital is concerned because the volume of remittance advice remark code #M39 (The patient is not liable for payment for this service as the advance notice of noncoverage you provided the patient did not comply with program requirements) on Medicare remittance advice logs has increased over the past 3 months. Further analysis of the denied claims shows that 75% of the claims have code 93798, Physician services for outpatient cardiac rehabilitation with continuous ECG monitoring, present. Therefore, they are requesting that the Revenue Cycle Team perform further investigation for this issue.

After auditing the remittance advice logs and medical records for a sample of cardiac rehabilitation claims, the Revenue Cycle Team has determined that medical necessity is not being met for code 93798. Further, they have discovered that a new LCD was issued for code 93798 in October (3 months ago). The only ICD-9-CM diagnosis codes that support medical necessity for code 93798 are:

- 410.00–410.92 Acute myocardial infarction of anterolateral wall episode of care unspecified through acute myocardial infarction of unspecified site subsequent episode of care
- Old myocardial infarction
- 413.0–413.9* Angina decubitus through other and unspecified angina pectoris
- V45.81 Post surgical aortocoronary bypass status

*There is no specific code assigned to stable angina. Therefore, these codes should be used to identify stable angina and documentation should support that diagnosis.

Further, around $20,790.00 has been written off due to ABNs not being issued for this cardiac rehabilitation service. Answer the following questions:

a. What went wrong in the revenue cycle?

b. How would you suggest rectifying this issue?

c. How will your team monitor improvements?

NOTE: Information for medical necessity/ABN example taken from LCD for Cardiac Rehabilitation Services L2650, which can be retrieved at www.cms.hhs.gov.

3. Review the following excerpt from the charge description master file at Anywhere Hospital. Closely examine the line items and identify and correct the elements that need to be updated or revised.

Item Code	Service Description	Revenue Code	CPT Code	Price
12345	BILIRUBIN TOTAL & DIRECT	310	82251	$25.00
12347	CHROMOSOME STUDY—AMNIOTIC FLUID	300		$0.00
12350	SKIN TEST CAND	300	86458	$20.00
12351	TRANSCATHETER PLACEMENT.IVSTENT VESSLE	320	95960	$1,125.00
12348	CT CHEST W/WO ABD&PELVIS W/CONTRAST	352		$1.00
12346	CATHETERIZATION URETHRA COMPLICATED	360	53675	$270.00
12349	OPERATING ROOM-III 1ST 30 MINUTES	360		$2,267.00
12352	HOT/COLD THERAPY PT	430		$75.00
12353	LEVEL 2 DRUG	250		$3,000.00

4. The executive finance team at Anywhere Hospital is reviewing charge levels for various surgical units. The team leader has requested a CDM management report from the CDM coordinator. She would like the report to include the Medicare reimbursement, cost, and profit for procedures performed during first quarter 2008. Additionally, she would like third party payer average reimbursement, cost, and profit for the same time period.

   Using the information in Table 4.1, complete the data elements provided in Table 4.2. The average reimbursement rate for all third party payers at Anywhere Hospital is 62 percent of billed charges. The outpatient ratio of cost to charge for revenue code 360 is 0.4043. The outpatient ratio of cost to charge for revenue code 320 is 0.5267. Is either of the payers profitable for Anytime Hospital in this outpatient surgical area?

Table 4.1

Charge Code	Code Description	CPT Code	Rev Code	Revenue Area	Charge	Medicare Vol	TPP Vol
49213	BIOPSY BREAST PERCUT W/ O IMAGING GUIDANCE	19100	360	1137	826.80	58	115
49214	BIOPSY OF BREAST, OPEN	19101	360	1137	3944.25	37	76
49215	BIOPSY BREAST, PERCUT, W IMAGING GUIDANCE	19102	360	1137	1359.48	87	112
49216	BIOPSY BREAST, PERCUT W DEVICE	19103	360	1137	2594.22	63	123
49217	CRYOSURG ABLATE FIBROADENOMA, EACH	19105	360	1137	6059.85	21	32
49218	NIPPLE EXPLORATION	19110	360	1137	3944.25	12	14
49219	EXCISE BREAST DUCT FISTULA	19112	360	1137	3944.25	14	17
49220	REMOVAL OF BREAST LESION	19120	360	1137	3944.25	76	87
49221	EXCISION, BREAST LESION	19125	360	1137	3944.25	45	90
49222	EXCISION, ADDL BREAST LESION	19126	360	1137	3944.25	36	54
49223	REMOVAL OF CHEST WALL LESION	19260	360	1137	3076.44	22	43
49224	PREOP PLACE NEEDLE LOCAL WIRE BREAST	19290	320	1196	65.00	43	98
49225	PREOP NEEDLE LOCALIZATION ADD'L LESIONS	19291	320	1196	65.00	10	65
49226	TISSUE MARKER PLACEMENT	19295	320	1196	65.00	17	24
49227	PLACE BALLOON CATHETER FOR RADIOELEMENT APP	19296	360	1137	10810.92	5	24
49228	PLACE BALLOON CATHETER WITH PART MASTECTOMY	19297	360	1137	10810.92	8	12
49229	PLACE BRACHYTHERAPY CATHETER	19298	360	1137	10810.92	10	32
49230	REMOVAL OF BREAST TISSUE	19300	360	1137	3944.25	21	68
49231	PARTIAL MASTECTOMY	19301	360	1137	3944.25	24	45

(Continued on next page)

Charge Code	Code Description	CPT Code	Rev Code	Revenue Area	Charge	Medicare Vol	TPP Vol
49232	P-MASTECTOMY W LYMPHADENECTOMY	19302	360	1137	7608.72	21	65
49233	MASTECTOMY, SIMPLE, COMPLETE	19303	360	1137	6059.85	18	47
49234	MASTECTOMY, SUBCUTANEOUS	19304	360	1137	6059.85	17	56
49235	MASTECTOMY, MODIFIED RADICAL	19307	360	1137	7608.72	15	63
49236	SUSPENSION OF BREAST	19316	360	1137	6059.85	11	2
49237	REDUCTION OF LARGE BREAST	19318	360	1137	7608.72	9	12
49238	ENLARGE BREAST	19324	360	1137	7608.72	0	23
49239	ENLARGE BREASE WITH IMPLANT	19325	360	1137	10810.92	0	25
49240	REMOVAL OF BREAST IMPLANT	19328	360	1137	6059.85	5	13
49241	REMOVAL OF BREAST IMPLANT MATERIAL	19330	360	1137	6059.85	0	16
49242	IMMEDIATE BREAST PROSTHESIS	19340	360	1137	7608.72	0	34
49243	DELAYED BREAST PROSTHESIS	19342	360	1137	10810.92	17	27
49244	BREAST RECONSTRUCTION	19350	360	1137	3944.25	4	47
49245	CORRECT INVERTED NIPPLE(S)	19355	360	1137	6059.85	0	3
49246	BREAST RECONSTRUCTION	19357	360	1137	10810.92	6	25
49247	BREAST RECONSTRUCTION	19366	360	1137	6059.85	7	24
49248	SURGERY OF BREAST CAPSULE	19370	360	1137	6059.85	5	12
49249	REMOVAL OF BREAST CAPSULE	19371	360	1137	6059.85	6	9
49250	REVISE BREAST RECONSTRUCTION	19380	360	1137	7608.72	4	8
49251	DESIGN CUSTOM BREAST IMPLANT	19396	360	1137	6059.85	0	23
49252	BREAST SURGERY PROCEDURE	19499	360	1137	3944.25	2	1

Table 4.2

Charge Code	Code Description	CPT Code	MCR Reimb	TPP Reimb	MCR Cost	TPP Cost	MCR Profit	TPP Profit
49213	BIOPSY BREAST PERCUT W/O IMAGING GUIDANCE	19100						
49214	BIOPSY OF BREAST, OPEN	19101						
49215	BIOPSY BREAST, PERCUT, W IMAGING GUIDANCE	19102						
49216	BIOPSY BREAST, PERCUT W DEVICE	19103						
49217	CRYOSURG ABLATE FIBROADENOMA, EACH	19105						
49218	NIPPLE EXPLORATION	19110						
49219	EXCISE BREAST DUCT FISTULA	19112						
49220	REMOVAL OF BREAST LESION	19120						
49221	EXCISION, BREAST LESION	19125						
49222	EXCISION, ADDL BREAST LESION	19126						
49223	REMOVAL OF CHEST WALL LESION	19260						
49224	PREOP PLACE NEEDLE LOCAL WIRE BREAST	19290						
49225	PREOP NEEDLE LOCALIZATION ADD'L LESIONS	19291						
49226	TISSUE MARKER PLACEMENT	19295						
49227	PLACE BALLOON CATHETER FOR RADIOELEMENT APP	19296						
49228	PLACE BALLOON CATHETER WITH PART MASTECTOMY	19297						
49229	PLACE BRACHYTHERAPY CATHETER	19298						
49230	REMOVAL OF BREAST TISSUE	19300						
49231	PARTIAL MASTECTOMY	19301						
49232	P-MASTECTOMY W LYMPHADENECTOMY	19302						
49233	MASTECTOMY, SIMPLE, COMPLETE	19303						
49234	MASTECTOMY, SUBCUTANEOUS	19304						
49235	MASTECTOMY, MODIFIED RADICAL	19307						
49236	SUSPENSION OF BREAST	19316						
49237	REDUCTION OF LARGE BREAST	19318						

(Continued on next page)

Charge Code	Code Description	CPT Code	MCR Reimb	TPP Reimb	MCR Cost	TPP Cost	MCR Profit	TPP Profit
49238	ENLARGE BREAST	19324						
49239	ENLARGE BREASE WITH IMPLANT	19325						
49240	REMOVAL OF BREAST IMPLANT	19328						
49241	REMOVAL OF BREAST IMPLANT MATERIAL	19330						
49242	IMMEDIATE BREAST PROSTHESIS	19340						
49243	DELAYED BREAST PROSTHESIS	19342						
49244	BREAST RECONSTRUCTION	19350						
49245	CORRECT INVERTED NIPPLE(S)	19355						
49246	BREAST RECONSTRUCTION	19357						
49247	BREAST RECONSTRUCTION	19366						
49248	SURGERY OF BREAST CAPSULE	19370						
49249	REMOVAL OF BREAST CAPSULE	19371						
49250	REVISE BREAST RECONSTRUCTION	19380						
49251	DESIGN CUSTOM BREAST IMPLANT	19396						
49252	BREAST SURGERY PROCEDURE	19499						

5. Identify five new CPT codes for the upcoming calendar year. Create a workflow to ensure that all data elements required in the CDM are identified, verified, and signed off on for inclusion in the CDM. Identify any compliance issues for these new CPT codes.

Review Quiz

1. Which provider order entry system is usually more reliable, paper-based or electronic? Why?
2. What are two sources of new charge description master codes?
3. What risk areas are concerns when the charge description master is not properly maintained and revised?
4. How has HIPAA changed claims processing?
5. What are two roles of EDI in claims processing?
6. List the ways discrepancies between submitted charges and paid charges are reconciled by the provider.
7. How do providers decide what optimal performance is for units of their facility?
8. Facility B just completed an analysis of its alarmingly high balance of unpaid claim amounts. What are some key performance indicators a provider's RCM team could use to learn the reason(s) for the surge in unpaid balances?
9. Describe at least three sources of errors that cause claim denials.
10. Use of the charge description master has made manual coding by HIM coders obsolete. True or false?

Chapter 9
Quality Issues

Theory into Practice

Pay-for-performance (P4P) systems are rapidly evolving across the healthcare sector. As these systems link reimbursement, performance, and quality, they tap into national trends for increased accountability and quality. As stated in the text, many models for P4P systems exist. In this discussion of theory into practice, we examine why.

Researchers examined the strategies, the development, and the implementation of P4P systems across several types of healthcare plans in twelve metropolitan areas (Trude et al. 2006, 537). The types of healthcare plans were Blue Cross and Blue Shield plans, national healthcare plans (such as Kaiser Permanente or the UnitedHealth Group), and a local healthcare plan (Trude et al. 2006, 538).

Strategies common across 77 percent of the P4P systems were hospital-based pay-for-performance or physician-based pay-for-performance. Across-the-board, the healthcare plans' representatives stated that their goal was to improve quality and provider efficiency and, thereby, reduce costs (Trude et al. 2006, 538). Thus, incentives could be categorized as (a) performing comparable with benchmarks, (b) achieving absolute targets, and (c) demonstrating improvement over past scores (Trude et al. 2006, 540).

Several variations, based on local conditions, were found. These local conditions included the providers' willingness to participate, the employers' interest and influence, the availability of data, the capabilities of health information technologies, and the relative power of providers and healthcare plans (Trude et al. 2006, 538). For example, the researchers explained that the "clout" of the Cleveland Clinic Health System limited the development of P4P systems in the Cleveland area (Trude et al. 2006, 539). In another instance, physicians in Syracuse were reluctant to invest in the health information technologies so the healthcare plans had targeted their P4P strategies at hospitals (Trude et al. 2006, 539).

A common problem was the development of performance measures. Providers wanted clinically valid measures. Some physicians added that they wanted the outcomes on performance measures to be within their control, such as dependent upon changes in the medical practice, and not dependent upon changes in patients' behavior. For example, in

Syracuse, many healthcare policies had high out-of-pocket costs for preventive care and patients often postponed preventive follow-ups. However, many P4P measures are based on levels of patient compliance with preventive care. These physicians felt they would be unfairly disadvantaged based on the design of the healthcare policies. In another metropolitan area, several healthcare plans implemented different performance measures. Providers interacting with these several healthcare plans had the administrative burden of collecting data for all the measures (Trude et al. 2006, 541).

Local customization and accommodation were common. Thus, the researchers concluded, that although national standardized measures could potentially increase efficiency, these measures may face local resistance because of the lack of local input (Trude et al. 2006, 542).

Reference

Trude, S., M. Au, and J.B. Christianson. 2006. Health plan pay-for-performance strategies. *American Journal of Managed Care* 12(9):537–542.

Real-World Case

Pay-for-performance (P4P) systems have existed in Medicaid since the early 2000s (Carlson 2000, n.p.). Given the emphasis on accountability across government programs, state Medicaid systems have continued to embrace this trend that links reimbursement, performance, and quality.

In 2006, over 50 percent of the 50 states' Medicaid programs included P4P systems or procedures. By 2011, if all planned P4P programs are implemented, almost 85 percent of states' Medicaid programs will include P4P (Kuhmerker and Hartman 2007a, viii).

Performance measures across the states' Medicaid plans vary widely (Kuhmerker and Hartman 2007a, 13). Often these performance measures are the Health Plan Employer Data and Information Set (HEDIS®) measures or a similar set (Kuhmerker and Hartman 2007a, 8). Included in the HEDIS are measures related to immunizations, screenings, appropriate prescriptions, and preventive and follow-up care (National Committee for Quality Assurance 2007, 1-1 to 1-11).

Meeting or exceeding the targets or thresholds in the performance measures is thought to represent quality and results rewards or penalties. The states' Medicaid programs have structured their financial incentives in many different ways.

References

Carlson, B. 2000, April. Many state Medicaid agencies use financial incentives to boost quality. *Managed Care* 9(4):13–14.

Gottschalk, A., and S.A. Flocke. 2005, November-December. Time spent in face-to-face patient care and work outside the examination room. *Annals of Family Medicine* 3(6):488–493.

Kuhmerker, K., and T. Hartman. 2007a, April. Pay-for-performance in state Medicaid programs: A survey of state Medicaid directors and programs. Available online from http://www.cmwf.org/publications/publications_show.htm?doc_id=472891. Accessed on 16 November 2007.

Kuhmerker, K., and T. Hartman. 2007b, April. Pay-for-performance in state Medicaid programs: A survey of state Medicaid directors and programs: Appendix B: State pay-for-performance program summaries. Available online from http://www.cmwf.org/publications/publications_show.htm?doc_id=472891. Accessed on 16 November 2007.

National Committee for Quality Assurance. 2007. HEDIS 2008 summary table of measures, product lines, and changes. Available online from http://web.ncqa.org/Portals/0/HEDISQM/HEDIS2008/2008_Measures.pdf. Accessed on 16 November 2007.

Questions

1. Has your state's Medicaid program implemented P4P (See Kuhmerker and Hartman 2007b, Appendix B, 1–82.)?
2. Does your state's Medicaid program plan to implement P4P (See Kuhmerker and Hartman 2007b, Appendix B, 1–82.)?
3. If your state's Medicaid program is one of the few that has not implemented or is not planning to implement P4P, do any of your neighboring states' Medicaid programs have P4P or plan to implement P4P (See Kuhmerker and Hartman 2007b, Appendix B, 1–82.)?

Application Activity for Real-World Case

Find your state's Medicaid program and use the components of its existing or planned P4P system to complete the following exercises. If your state's Medicaid program is one of the few that has not implemented P4P and does not plan to implement P4P, select a neighboring state for these exercises. See Kuhmerker and Hartman 2007b, Appendix B, 1-82.

1. Which providers are targeted by P4P?
2. What is the type of incentive and its methodology?
3. What are its measures?
4. Does the P4P system use the HEDIS® measures? See the list of the HEDIS® measures at the Web site of the National Committee for Quality Assurance http://web.ncqa.org/Portals/0/HEDISQM/HEDIS2008/2008_Measures.pdf.
5. Scenario. A family physician sees approximately 29 patients per day (Gottschalk and Flocke 2005, 490–491). Of these 29 patients per day, 5 are Medicaid patients and 3 of those Medicaid patients are well babies. The state Medicaid plan has implemented P4P and is utilizing the HEDIS® measures. One of the measures is that well babies have 6 office visits by 15 months. At the current time, the family physician receives a $100 bonus per baby with 6 or more well-baby visits by 15 months. The Medicaid program has proposed two methods of restructuring the incentives:

- $25 bonus for each set of 3 well-baby visits to the family physician and a $15 gift certificate for each set of 2 well-baby visits to the parents
- $100 bonus per baby receiving fifth well-baby visit and polio, hepatitis B, and Haemophilus influenzae type b (Hib) vaccines by 13 months and a second $100 bonus for the sixth well-baby visit by 15 months and relevant vaccines

Of the three methods, current and two proposed, which method would result in the highest financial reward for the family physician? Which method would result in the lowest financial reward for the family physician?

Application Exercises

1. CMS is adding pay-for-performance provisions to their prospective payment systems. The Hospital Acquired Conditions provision will take effect in FY 2009 for IPPS; Medicare payments will be reduced starting October 1, 2008. Under this provision, the quality of care provided to the Medicare beneficiary is determined by what is documented in the medical record, i.e. was the condition acquired during the hospital admission or was it present when the patient was admitted to the hospital for inpatient services. Therefore, physician documentation is the key. Prepare an educational presentation regarding this provision for your Medical Director and Department Heads. The presentation should highlight the importance of accurate and timely physician documentation. Provide examples of how this provision may affect Medicare reimbursement. Also, consider how delayed documentation could affect the number of days in "discharged not final billed"—how does this affect the financial position of the hospital?

2. Under the Hospital Acquired Conditions provision of the IPPS, the Secretary of Health and Human Services has designated several conditions that when acquired during a hospital admission have the potential to reduce MS-DRG payment. One of the conditions applicable for FY 2009 is pressure ulcers (ICD-9-CM codes 707.0X). To identify if the pressure ulcer was present when the patient was admitted or was acquired during the hospital stay, the hospital must report a present-on-admission code for each diagnosis on the UB-04 form.

   Scenario: Stephanie is the coding manager at Anywhere Hospital. The coders have been charged with applying the present-on-admission indicator code. Stephanie has collected data over the past six months. It is quite clear from the data that there is an issue with either the documentation of pressure ulcers, assignment of the POA indicator, or the quality of care provided at Anywhere Hospital. Stephanie has requested that Sally, one of the Quality Managers, assist her with this issue.

POA Report for Pressure Ulcers (707.0x) October–March

POA Code	Description	Volume
Y	Yes, present on admission	15
N	No, not present on admission	30
U	Unknown, insufficient documentation	45
W	Clinically undetermined	3
1	Exempt from POA reporting	0

It is clear that a medical record audit is necessary to determine if there is a documentation, POA assignment, or quality of care issue. ***Design an audit plan for this issue.*** What questions should be asked? What processes need to be examined? Who should conduct the audit?

3. Research the *Physician Group Practice (PGP) Demonstration* project sponsored by the Centers for Medicare and Medicaid Services. Start with the CMS Web site at www.cms.hhs.gov.
   a. What are the goals of the demonstration?
   b. What quality measures are utilized in this demonstration?
   c. Which ten physician groups are participating in this demonstration?
   d. What incentive structure is used to influence the physician groups to improve the quality of care provided to their Medicare patients?
   e. What are the results so far?

Review Quiz

1. What three components do pay-for-performance systems typically link?
2. Why did pay-for-performance systems emerge?
3. What incentives are typically aligned in pay-for-performance systems?
4. The very first pay-for-performance systems emerged in the early 1990s. True or False?
5. The Centers for Medicare and Medicaid Services has attempted to brake the trend to pay-for-performance systems because its experts believe the linkage of quality and rewards jeopardizes the care of patients. True or False?
6. List three other countries that are investigating pay-for-performance systems for their healthcare delivery systems.

7. Withholding compensation would be considered a penalty-based model of pay-for-performance. True or False?
8. CMS has established one value-based purchasing demonstration project and it is for the hospital inpatient setting. True or False?
9. What clinical areas are included in the Premier Hospital Quality Incentive Demonstration (HQID)?
10. Under the Reporting of Hospital Quality Data for Annual Payment Update (RHQDAPU) program, hospitals have to demonstrate that the quality of care has improved at their facility in order to achieve and/or maintain the annual payment update percentage. True or False?

Answer Sheets

Name: ______________________________

Section: ____________________________

Answer Sheet for Chapter 1

Questions

1. ____

2. ____

____

3. ____

____

Application Exercises

2. ____

____

____

3. ________

4. ____

____

____

Review Quiz

1. ____

____

____

2. ____

____

____

3. ____

____

____

(Attach additional sheet if necessary.)

4. ____

____

____

5. ____

____

____

6. ____

____

____

7. ____

____

____

8. ____

____

____

9. __________

10. ____

____

____

Name: ______________________

Section: ______________________

Answer Sheet for Chapter 2

Application Exercises

1. ______________________

2. ______________________

3. ______________________

Review Quiz

1. ________

2. ________

3. ________

4. ________

5. ______________________

6. ______________________

7. ______________________

(Attach additional sheet if necessary.)

8. ____

____

____

9. ____

10. ____

11. ____

____

12. ____

13. ____

____

14. ____

____

____

15. ____

16. ________

17. ________

18. ________

19. ________

Name: ______________________________

Section: ______________________________

Answer Sheet for Chapter 3

Questions

1. ________

2. ____

3. ____

   ____

   ____

4. ____

   ____

   ____

5. ____

   ____

   ____

6. ________

(Attach additional sheet if necessary.)

Application Exercises

2. ____

____

____

3.

Comparison: Out-of-Pocket Costs by Healthcare Insurance Company

Type of Cost	Example	Healthcare Co. A	Healthcare Co. B	Healthcare Co. C	Healthcare Co. D
Annual Premium (Monthly × 12)	\$56 × 12 = \$672 (Individual)				
Annual Deductibles	\$350 per Covered Individual				
Drugs	\$0				
Physician Office Visits	Inc. in \$350				
Inpatient	Inc. in \$350				
Outpatient	Inc. in \$350				
Mental Health	Inc. in \$350				
Outpatient Therapy (PT, OT, Speech)	Inc. in \$350				
Chiropractic	Inc. in \$350				
Other					
Copayments					
Dental	\$15 per Visit for Accident, Routine Not Covered				
Drugs	Each 34-Day Supply: \$10 Generic, \$25 Preferred Brand without Generic, \$40 Preferred Brand with Generic, \$50 Non-Preferred Brand (\$10 Generic × 12 mos. = \$120)				
Physician Office Visits	\$15 per Visit (\$15 × 4 Visits per Year = \$60)				
Inpatient	\$150 per Admission				

(Continued on next answer sheet)

Name: ______________________

Section: ______________________

Answer Sheet for Chapter 3 (Continued)

Type of Cost	Example	Healthcare Co. A	Healthcare Co. B	Healthcare Co. C	Healthcare Co. D
Mental Health	$150 Inpatient Care, $15 per Visit, $100 Treatment Admission				
Outpatient Therapy (PT, OT, Speech)	$15 per Visit				
Chiropractic	$15 per Visit				
Outpatient Hospital or Amb. Surg.	$75 per Episode				
Emergency Room	$200 per Visit (Unless Admitted)				
Vision	$15 per Medical Eye Exam, Glasses etc. Not Covered				
Other					
Coinsurance	20% up to $2,000 per Member				
Inpatient	See 20% above				
Outpatient	See 20% above				
Other					
Ambulance	Prior Approval				
Home Care	Prior Approval				
Private Duty Nurse	Prior Approval				
SNF	Prior Approval				
Other Out-of-Pocket					
TOTAL	**$1,202 before Lab Work or X-rays (4 clinic visits and generic meds)**				

(Attach additional sheet if necessary.)

Review Quiz

1. ____
____
____

2. ____
____
____

3. ____
____
____

4. ____
____
____

5. ____
____
____

6. ____
____
____

7. ____
____
____

8. ________

9. ________

10. ________

Name: ______________________________

Section: ______________________________

Answer Sheet for Chapter 4

Application Exercises

2. ______________________________

Review Quiz

1. ______________________________
2. ______________________________
3. ______________________________
4. ______________________________
5. ______________________________

(Attach additional sheet if necessary.)

6. ____

____

____

7. ____

8. ________

9. ________

10. ________

Name: ____________________

Section: ____________________

Answer Sheet for Chapter 5

Questions

1. ________
2. ____________________
3. ____________________
4. ____________________

Application Exercises

3. ____________________
4. ____________________

Review Quiz

1. ____________________

(Attach additional sheet if necessary.)

2. ____

____

____

3. ____

____

____

____

____

____

4. ____

____

____

5. ____

____

____

6. ____

7. ____

____

8. ________

9. ________

10. ________

Name: ______________________

Section: ______________________

Answer Sheet for Chapter 6

Application Exercises

1. ____

____

2. ____

____

3.

	2 Years Ago	1 Year Ago	Current Year
Year			
Local Wage Index			
Standard Payment Conversion Factor			
Impact of Change in Wage Index (+ or –) Per Case			
Multiplied by No. of Discharges Annually (Ex: 370)			

4.

Table 1

Step	Methodology	Total
One	(per-diem rate × .75788 × WI)	
Two	If COLA then (per-diem rate ×.24212 × COLA) If non-COLA then (per-diem rate × .24212)	
Three	Sum results of step 1 and step 2	
Four	Use mini-worksheet A (see below)	
Five	Multiply result of step 3 times result of step 4	
Six	If full service ED then choose higher Day 1 adjustment in step 7 If not full service ED then choose lower Day 1 adjustment in step 7	
Seven	Use mini-worksheet B (see below)	
Eight	Sum of day rates calculated in step 7	
Nine	If COLA then ((ECT pymt rate × .75788 × WI)+(ECT pymt rate × .24212 × COLA)) × units of service If non-COLA then ((ECT pymt rate × .75788 × WI) + (ECT pymt rate × .24212)) × units of service	
Ten	Sum results of step 8 and 9	

(Attach additional sheet if necessary.)

Mini Worksheet A			
Step Four	A. Enter adjustment factor if rural location:		Enter PPS adjustment factor in Table 1 row four.
	B. Enter adjustment factor if teaching facility:		
	C. Enter adjustment factor for DRG:		
	D. Enter adjustment factor for comorbidity:		
	E. Enter adjustment factor for age:		
	Multiply applicable adjustment factors together to determine PPS adjustment factor:		

Mini Worksheet B			
Step Seven	**Day**	**Adjustment Factor**	**Adj. Factor × adjusted per-diem rate (step 5)**
	Day one		
	Day two		
	Day three		
	Day four		
	Day five		
	Day six		
	Day seven		
	Day eight		
	Day nine		
	Day ten		
	Day eleven		
	Day twelve		
	Day thirteen		
	Day fourteen		

5. ____

____

Name: ____________________

Section: ____________________

Answer Sheet for Chapter 6 (Continued)

Review Quiz

1. ____________________
____
____
____

2. ____________________
____
____

3. ____________________
____
____

4. ____________________

5. ____________________
____
____

6. ____________________

7. ____________________
____
____

8. ________

9. ________

(Attach additional sheet if necessary.)

Name: ______________________

Section: ______________________

Answer Sheet for Chapter 7

Questions

1. ______________________

2. ______________________

3. ______________________

Application Exercises

1. ______________________

2. ______________________

3a. ______________________

(Attach additional sheet if necessary.)

3b.

Weight 1.9413	Nat'l 60-day episode rate (CY current) ($)	Unadjusted rate ($)	Labor-related ratio	Local wage index	Adj labor portion (unadj. rate × labor ratio × local wage index)	Non-labor related ratio	Unadjusted nonlabor portion (unadj. rate × nonlabor ratio)	Wage adj. rate (adj. labor portion + unadj. nonlabor ratio) ($)

3c.

National Per-Visit Amounts for LUPAs by Discipline (Not Including A Beneficiary's Only Episode or the Initial Episode in a Sequence of Adjacent Episodes)*

Home Health Discipline Type	Per-Visit Payment Amount CY Current Year
Home Health Aide	
Medical Social Services	
Occupational Therapy	
Physical Therapy	
Skilled Nursing	
Speech-Language Pathology	

*Modified Source: *Federal Register* 70(216) p. 68134.

Department of Health and Human Services. 2005 (November 9). Medicare Program; Home Health Prospective Payment System Rate Update for Calendar Year 2006; Final Rule. *Federal Register* 70(216):68132–68215.

4.

Table 1

Step	Methodology	Total
One	APC relative weight × conversion factor ($63.694)	
Two	(APC pymt rate × .60×WI) + (APC pymt rate × .40)	
Three	Fee schedule amount A + fee schedule amount B, etc.	
Four	(Charge × CCR)	
Five	Total Reimbursement – Sum of steps 2–4	

Table 2

Step	Methodology	Total
One	APC relative weight × conversion factor ($41.401)	
Two	(APC pymt rate × .50*WI) + (APC pymt rate × .50)	
Three	APC relative weight × conversion factor ($41.401)	
Four	(APC pymt rate × .50*WI) + (APC pymt rate × .50)	
Five	TOTAL Reimbursement – Sum of steps 2–4	

Name: ______________________________

Section: ______________________________

Answer Sheet for Chapter 7 (Continued)

Short Discussion Question

Review Quiz

1.

2.

3.

4.

5.

(Attach additional sheet if necessary.)

6. __________

7. ____

____

____

8. __________

9. __________

10. __________

Name: ______________________________

Section: ____________________________

Answer Sheet for Chapter 8

Questions

1. ______________________________
____
____

2. ______________________________
____
____

3. ______________________________
____
____

Application Exercise

1a. ______________________________
____

1b. ______________________________
____

1c. ______________________________
____

1d. ______________________________
____

2a. ______________________________
____
____

2b. ______________________________
____
____

(Attach additional sheet if necessary.)

2c. ____

____

____

3.

Item Code	Service Description	Revenue Code	CPT Code	Price
12345	BILIRUBIN TOTAL & DIRECT	310	82251	$25.00
12347	CHROMOSOME STUDY—AMNIOTIC FLUID	300		$0.00
12350	SKIN TEST CAND	300	86458	$20.00
12351	TRANSCATHETER PLACEMENT.IVSTENT VESSLE	320	95960	$1,125.00
12348	CT CHEST W/WO ABD&PELVIS W/CONTRAST	352		$1.00
12346	CATHETERIZATION URETHRA COMPLICATED	360	53675	$270.00
12349	OPERATING ROOM-III 1ST 30 MINUTES	360		$2,267.00
12352	HOT/COLD THERAPY PT	430		$75.00
12353	LEVEL 2 DRUG	250		$3,000.00

4.

Charge Code	Code Description	CPT Code	MCR Reimb	TPP Reimb	MCR Cost	TPP Cost	MCR Profit	TPP Profit
49213	BIOPSY BREAST PERCUT W/O IMAGING GUIDANCE	19100						
49214	BIOPSY OF BREAST, OPEN	19101						
49215	BIOPSY BREAST, PERCUT, W IMAGING GUIDANCE	19102						
49216	BIOPSY BREAST, PERCUT W DEVICE	19103						
49217	CRYOSURG ABLATE FIBROADENOMA, EACH	19105						
49218	NIPPLE EXPLORATION	19110						
49219	EXCISE BREAST DUCT FISTULA	19112						
49220	REMOVAL OF BREAST LESION	19120						
49221	EXCISION, BREAST LESION	19125						
49222	EXCISION, ADDL BREAST LESION	19126						
49223	REMOVAL OF CHEST WALL LESION	19260						
49224	PREOP PLACE NEEDLE LOCAL WIRE BREAST	19290						
49225	PREOP NEEDLE LOCALIZATION ADD'L LESIONS	19291						
49226	TISSUE MARKER PLACEMENT	19295						

Name: ____________________

Section: ____________________

Answer Sheet for Chapter 8 (Continued)

Charge Code	Code Description	CPT Code	MCR Reimb	TPP Reimb	MCR Cost	TPP Cost	MCR Profit	TPP Profit
49227	PLACE BALLOON CATHETER FOR RADIOELEMENT APP	19296						
49228	PLACE BALLOON CATHETER WITH PART MASTECTOMY	19297						
49229	PLACE BRACHYTHERAPY CATHETER	19298						
49230	REMOVAL OF BREAST TISSUE	19300						
49231	PARTIAL MASTECTOMY	19301						
49232	P-MASTECTOMY W LYMPHADENECTOMY	19302						
49233	MASTECTOMY, SIMPLE, COMPLETE	19303						
49234	MASTECTOMY, SUBCUTANEOUS	19304						
49235	MASTECTOMY, MODIFIED RADICAL	19307						
49236	SUSPENSION OF BREAST	19316						
49237	REDUCTION OF LARGE BREAST	19318						
49238	ENLARGE BREAST	19324						
49239	ENLARGE BREASE WITH IMPLANT	19325						
49240	REMOVAL OF BREAST IMPLANT	19328						
49241	REMOVAL OF BREAST IMPLANT MATERIAL	19330						
49242	IMMEDIATE BREAST PROSTHESIS	19340						
49243	DELAYED BREAST PROSTHESIS	19342						
49244	BREAST RECONSTRUCTION	19350						
49245	CORRECT INVERTED NIPPLE(S)	19355						
49246	BREAST RECONSTRUCTION	19357						
49247	BREAST RECONSTRUCTION	19366						
49248	SURGERY OF BREAST CAPSULE	19370						
49249	REMOVAL OF BREAST CAPSULE	19371						
49250	REVISE BREAST RECONSTRUCTION	19380						
49251	DESIGN CUSTOM BREAST IMPLANT	19396						
49252	BREAST SURGERY PROCEDURE	19499						

(Attach additional sheet if necessary.)

5. ______________________________

Review Quiz

1. ______________________________

2. ______________________________

3. ______________________________

4. ______________________________

5. ______________________________

6. ______________________________

7. ______________________________

8. ______________________________

9. ______________________________

10. __________

Name: ______________________________

Section: ____________________________

Answer Sheet for Chapter 9

Questions

1. ________

2. ________

3. ________

Application Activity for Real-World Case

1. ____

____

2. ____

____

____

3. ____

____

____

4. ________

5. ____

____

____

Application Exercises

2. ____

____

____

(Attach additional sheet if necessary.)

3a. ______________________________

____

____

3b. ______________________________

____

____

3c. ______________________________

____

____

3d. ______________________________

____

____

3e. ______________________________

____

____

Review Quiz

1. ______________________________

____

____

2. ______________________________

____

____

3. ______________________________

____

____

4. ________

5. ________

6. ______________________________

____

____

Name: ______________________________

Section: ____________________________

Answer Sheet for Chapter 9 (Continued)

7. ________

8. ________

9. ____

   ____

   ____

10. ________

(Attach additional sheet if necessary.)

NOTES